REDUCE ANXIENTY: THE COMPLETE

GUIDE ON XANAX

The Step-By-Step Guide for The Treatment of Panic Disorder, And Anxiety Disorders, Such as Generalized Anxiety Disorder or Social Anxiety Disorder.

ISBN 978-1-6780-3425-2

Rylan Peterson

TABLE OF CONTENT

WHAT EXACTLY IS XANAX?

Xanax (alprazolam) is a benzodiazepine that is used to treat anxiety (ben-zoe-dye-AZE-eh-peen). Several neurotransmitters in the brain are thought to be involved in alprazolam's action, which is thought to be the case.

Xanax is a prescription medication that is used to treat anxiety disorders and anxiety caused by depression.

Xanax is also used to treat panic disorders, which can include a fear of places and situations that cause panic, helplessness, or embarrassment. Xanax is also used to treat anxiety disorders (agoraphobia).

Purchasing Xanax via the Internet or from a source outside of the United States is extremely dangerous. The sale and distribution of pharmaceuticals outside of the United States does not conform with the Food and Drug Administration's laws on safe use of medications (FDA). These prescriptions may include potentially hazardous substances, or they may not be distributed by a licensed pharmacy in the first instance.

WARNINGS

If you have recently used an opioid medicine or consumed alcohol, Xanax may cause your breathing to become more difficult or impossible to control.

Addiction, overdose, and death can result from the improper use of XANAX. Keep the medication in a secure location where others will not be able to get it.

Do not discontinue Xanax use without first consulting your doctor. If you suddenly stop taking the medication after a long period of time, you may experience life-threatening withdrawal symptoms. Some withdrawal symptoms can linger for up to 12 months or longer in some cases.

If you suddenly stop taking Xanax and experience symptoms such as strange muscular movements, becoming more energetic or talkative, sudden and severe changes in mood or behavior, confusion, hallucinations, seizures, or thoughts of suicide, seek medical attention right away.

Xanax is classified as a Schedule IV controlled substance (C-IV) by the federal government because it has the potential to be abused or to induce dependence. This medication should be stored in a secure location to avoid overuse and abuse. Selling or giving away this Xanax may cause harm to others and is therefore prohibited by law. Please inform your healthcare practitioner if you have used alcohol, prescription medications, or street drugs and have become addicted to them.

Prior to taking this medication, you should consult your doctor.

If you have any of the following symptoms, you should not take Xanax:

In addition, you may be taking antifungal medications such as itraconazole or ketoconazole.

have a history of allergic reactions to benzodiazepines in the past (alprazolam, lorazepam, diazepam, Ativan, Valium, Versed, Klonopin, and others).

Before taking Xanax, tell your doctor about any medical conditions you have had in the past.

- an issue with one's breathing;

- Addiction to drugs or alcohol;

- sadness, mood difficulties, or suicidal thoughts or conduct; or a combination of the above.

- Disease of the kidneys or liver

Inform your doctor if you are expecting a child or if you intend to become pregnant. It is possible that your baby will be delivered with life-threatening withdrawal symptoms if you use Xanax during pregnancy, and that he or she will require medical attention for several weeks.

It is not recommended that you breastfeed.

If you breastfeed your child, notify your doctor if you observe drowsiness or feeding difficulties in the child.

Anyone under the age of eighteen (18) is not permitted to use this product.

What is the best way to take Xanax?

Make sure to take Xanax exactly as your doctor has instructed. Follow the recommendations on your prescription label and be sure to read any medication guides or instruction sheets that come with your medication. Never take Xanax in greater doses or for a longer period of time than advised. Inform your doctor if you notice a sudden rise in the desire to take more of this medication.

This medication should never be shared with anyone else, especially with someone who has a history of drug abuse or addiction. Addiction, overdose, and even death can result from improper use. Keep the medication in a secure location where others will not be able to get it. It is against the law to sell or give away this prescription medication.

Take the extended-release pill of Xanax XR whole, without chewing or swallowing. This medication should not be crushed, chewed, or broken.

If your symptoms do not improve or if they worsen, you should consult your doctor.

If you use this medication for an extended period of time, you may require frequent medical examinations.

Do not discontinue Xanax use without first consulting your doctor. If you suddenly stop taking the medication after a long period of time, you may experience life-threatening withdrawal symptoms.

The medication should be stored at room temperature away from moisture, heat, and light. Keep your medication in a secure location where no one else can access it.

DOSAGE AND ADMINISTRATION INFORMATION

The usual adult dose for anxiety is:

Immediate-release tablets: 0.25 to 0.5 mg orally delivered three times.

- Maximum dose: 4 mg/day

The typical adult dose for panic disorder is as follows:

immediate-release tablets: Aim for a maximum daily dose of 10 mg using (0.5 mg orally delivered three times each day).

Extended-release time:

To begin, take between 0.5 and 1 mg orally once a day.

To maintain, take 3 to 6 mg orally once a day, preferably in the morning.

Maximum dose: 10 mg/day

Comments:

- The smallest effective dose should be supplied, and the need for continuing treatment should be evaluated on a regular basis.

- When terminating medication or decreasing the daily dosage, it is recommended that the dosage be reduced gradually.

If necessary, the daily dosage may be reduced by no more than 0.5 mg every 3 days; however, some patients may require a dosage reduction that is even more gradual.

In order to avoid overdosing on extended-release tablets, the dose should be raised at intervals between 3 and 4 days in increments of no more than 1 mg per day.

-The administration of medications should be spread out as equally as possible during the day's awake hours, according to the guidelines.

Anxiety in the Geriatric Population is usually treated with the following dosage:

Patients that are elderly or disabled:

The following dosage is for immediate-release tablets:

Initial dose: 0.25 mg orally delivered twice or three times per day.

The typical geriatric dose for panic disorder is as follows:

Patients that are elderly or disabled:

Tablets with an immediate release:

-Initial dose: 0.25 mg orally delivered twice or three times per day for the first week.

Tablets with a prolonged release time:

-Initial dose: 0.5 mg orally once a day for the first week

Observations:

-If there are any side effects, the dose may be reduced.

- In order to ensure that the smallest effective dose is delivered, the requirement for continuing treatment should be evaluated on a regular basis.

-When quitting therapy or reducing the daily dosage, it is best to reduce the dosage gradually to avoid side effects.

What happens if I don't take my medication on time?

Take the medication as soon as you are able, but if it is almost time for your next dose, omit the missed dose and continue with your regular schedule. Do not take more than one dose at a time.

What happens if I take too much or overdose?

Seek immediate medical attention or dial 1-800-222-1222 to reach the Poison Help hotline for assistance. An overdose of alprazolam can be lethal if taken with alcohol, opioid medication, or other substances that cause drowsiness or impede your breathing, as this is the case with many people.

Extreme drowsiness, disorientation, slurred speech, weakening of the muscles, loss of balance or coordination, feeling light-headed, slow heartbeats, weak or shallow breathing, fainting, or coma are all possible symptoms of an overdose.

WHAT TO AVOID

If I'm on Xanax, what should I stay away from?

Avoid consuming alcoholic beverages. It is possible that dangerous side effects or death will occur.

Avoid driving or engaging in other potentially dangerous activities until you know how this medication may effect you. Falls, accidents, and severe injuries can occur as a result of dizziness or drowsiness.

SIDE EFFECTS OF TAKING XANAX

If you see any of the following indicators of an allergic response to Xanax, seek immediate medical attention: Hives, difficulty breathing, swelling of the cheeks, lips, tongue, or throat are all possible symptoms.

Alprazolam can cause your breathing to become slowed or stopped, especially if you have recently used an opiate medicine or consumed alcohol. If you have slow breathing with extended pauses, bluish tinted lips, or if you are difficult to rouse up, someone caring for you should seek immediate medical treatment.

If you develop any of the following symptoms, call your doctor right away:

breathing that is feeble or shallow.

sensation of being dizzy and on the verge of passing out.

- a convulsion.

- hallucinations, and a tendency to take risks.

- decreased need for sleep due to enhanced energy levels

- race through one's thoughts, become anxious or chatty.

- double vision.

- Jaundice (yellowing of the skin or eyes).

In older adults, drowsiness or dizziness may linger for a longer period of time in older adults. Precaution should be exercised to avoid falling or suffering an unintended harm.

The following are some of the most common Xanax adverse effects:

- Sleepiness; or
- dizziness.

If you have any of the following symptoms after you stop taking Xanax: odd muscular movements, becoming more energetic or talkative, sudden and severe changes in mood or behavior, confusion, hallucinations, seizures, or suicidal thoughts or actions, seek medical attention as soon as possible.

It is possible that certain withdrawal symptoms will remain for up to 12 months or more after quitting this medication abruptly. Inform your doctor if you are experiencing persistent anxiety, depression, memory or thinking issues, difficulty sleeping, ringing in your ears, a burning or prickly sensation, or a crawling sensation beneath your skin.

The following is not a comprehensive list of possible side effects, and others may occur. For medical advice about side effects, consult with your doctor. You can report side effects to the Food and Drug Administration at 1-800-FDA-1088.

WHAT OTHER MEDICATIONS WILL HAVE AN EFFECT ON XANAX?

Using certain medications at the same time is not always a safe combination of actions. Some medications can have an influence on the levels of other medications in your blood, which can result in an increase in side effects or a decrease in the effectiveness of the medications.

Taking Xanax with other medications that make you sleepy or decrease your breathing might result in hazardous adverse effects or even death if used together. Before taking an opioid pain reliever, a sleeping pill, a muscle relaxer, or anything for anxiety or seizures, consult with your doctor.

Many medications can interact with alprazolam, and some medications should not be taken at the same time as alprazolam. Inform your doctor of any other medications you are taking. This covers prescription and over-the-counter medications, vitamins, and herbal supplements, among other things. Not all of the possible interactions are covered in this section.

Interactions between Xanax (alprazolam) with alcohol and food.

There are two types of alcohol/food/lifestyle interactions with Xanax (alprazolam), and they are as follows:

1. ALPRAZolam interacts with food in a moderate way.

Grapefruit and grapefruit juice have the potential to interact with ALPRAZolam, resulting in possibly harmful side effects. Consult your doctor about the consumption of grapefruit products. If you want to increase or decrease the amount of grapefruit products you consume, consult with your doctor first. ALPRAZolam should not be consumed with alcoholic beverages. This drug has the potential to enhance the effects of alcohol. If you combine

ALPRAZolam with alcohol, you may have increased drowsiness, dizziness, or fatigue. If you have any questions or concerns, you should consult your doctor or pharmacist.

2. Obesity

Potential danger is moderate, and believability is moderate.

Obesity is associated with benzodiazepines.

The half-lives of benzodiazepines in the plasma of obese persons may be prolonged, probably as a result of enhanced distribution into adipose tissue. For diazepam and midazolam, significant increases in distribution (more than 100 percent) have been recorded, whereas modest increases (ranging from 25 percent to 100 percent) have been documented for alprazolam, lorazepam, and oxazepam. Therapy with benzodiazepines should be delivered with caution in obese patients, and the patient's central nervous system should be closely monitored. It is possible that longer dose intervals will be necessary. For the purposes of avoiding toxicity, loading dosages should be calculated based on actual body weight, whereas maintenance doses should be calculated based on optimal body weight.

The disease interactions (9).

Xanax (alprazolam) Diseases Interactions.

Xanax (alprazolam) has nine(9) illness interactions that have been identified:

- Intoxication due to alcohol in a short period of time

- Glaucoma with a narrowed angle of vision

- Addiction to drugs

- Disease of the kidneys and liver

- Depression of the respiratory system

- Seizures

- Depression

- Obesity

- Reactions that are paradoxical

Acute alcohol intoxication caused by benzodiazepines (this includes Xanax). It is a major potential hazard with a high probability of occurring.

The use of benzodiazepines in conjunction with alcohol is not advised. Patients who are suffering from acute alcohol intoxication have lowered vital signs. A combination of benzodiazepines and alcohol may have additive depressive effects on the central nervous system, resulting in severe respiratory depression and mortality in certain instances. When administering benzodiazepines to individuals who are at risk for acute alcohol consumption, caution should be exercised in their administration.

How to Prevent a Fatal Drug Interaction:
The Top 9 Tips.

Because of the likelihood of a drug interaction, you should not be scared to take your prescription as prescribed. Drug interactions can be frightening for anyone who takes prescription prescriptions on a regular basis, but it is possible to learn how to manage and prevent these interactions.

Important medication interactions can occur with drugs that have a narrow therapeutic index (that is, where there is little difference between toxic and therapeutic doses) and with particular illness conditions such as epilepsy or depression. Additionally, when a person is taking many medications, as is frequently the situation with elderly patients, a number of drug interactions may arise.

However, while the majority of pharmaceutical interactions are not life threatening, some combinations of medications can have catastrophic — and even fatal — repercussions. Drug interactions are reviewed and predicted by pharmacists and doctors who have received extensive training. You can also utilize online medication interaction tools to assist you assess the risk of a drug interaction before consulting with your physician or pharmacist. As is always the case, if you have any questions, you should consult with your healthcare professional.

Educating and communicating with others are essential. In order to get the most out of your medical treatments, you should talk with your health-care providers, read only reputable drug information produced by professionals, and educate yourself on how to reduce the likelihood of drug interactions.

Here are nine suggestions to help you attain your objective.

1. Communicate with others on a regular basis.

Inform your pharmacist every time you begin or stop taking a medicine, including any over-the-counter (OTC) medication, herbal supplement, or vitamin supplement. Maintain an up-to-date list of medications — including over-the-counter medications — and share it with your health-care providers, including your doctor, pharmacist, and dentist, if you begin or discontinue taking a new medication.

Prescription medications are not the only medications that can interact with one another. Non-prescription medications, including over-the-counter medications, can have dangerous repercussions. For example, the herbal supplement St. John's Wort is frequently prescribed as an over-the-counter (OTC) treatment for depression. It is possible to develop a rare but serious and potentially fatal condition known as serotonin syndrome if antidepressants like fluoxetine (Prozac) or sertraline (Zoloft) are taken together. Symptoms include confusion, hallucinations, seizures, extreme blood pressure changes, and even death if the two antidepressants are taken together.

Every time you receive a new medication or a refill, make sure to read your Medication Guide and prescription labeling. The Food and Medicine Administration (FDA) updates prescription drug information on a regular basis, so there may be changes in your Medication Guide. Examine your potential interactions and feel free to ask questions if you are concerned or don't grasp the medical lingo completely.

Immediately notify your doctor if you discover that you are at risk for an interaction. It is possible that the interaction is insignificant and that no action is required. It is possible that you will need to avoid the pill or that you will be provided an alternate medication. Never discontinue taking a medication without first consulting your doctor.

2. Conduct your own research into your medication.

Become more involved in your health by using a dependable and user-friendly online drug interaction tool such as the Drugs.com

Interaction Checker to discover more about your drugs and become more active in your health. If you require assistance in comprehending the information, contact your pharmacist immediately. Even when purchasing over-the-counter drugs, herbal supplements, or vitamins, always sure to check for drug interactions.

For each drug interaction, the Drug Interaction Checker describes how it works, what its importance is (major, moderate, or minor), and in certain circumstances, it can prescribe a course of action to take to deal with it. If there are any interactions between your chosen drugs, food or beverages (such alcohol or grapefruit juice, which are both popular culprits), or even illness conditions, the Drug Interaction Checker will show you what they are.

Simply enter one drug name and click "Check for Interactions" to view all of the possible drug interactions that could occur. All interactions involving that medicine, both at the consumer and professional levels, are covered in detail in this section. If necessary, you or your healthcare practitioner can obtain professional recommendations from other professionals. You can also type in other drug names to check for interactions between two, three, or even more drugs at the same time.

3. Have all of your prescriptions filled at the same pharmacy.

By having all of your prescriptions filled at the same pharmacy, you can have a regular drug review and drug interaction screen performed electronically, which will include all of your medications. Consult with your pharmacist and doctor, and inform all of your health-care providers about any new or discontinued medications you may be taking. When it comes to preventing drug interactions, communication is essential.

When you purchase over-the-counter medications or herbal supplements, ask your pharmacist to double-check for drug interactions, and ask if the agent may be included to your normal drug profile so that future drug interaction tests can be performed. If your pharmacist is unaware that you are taking over-the-counter medications, they will be unable to check for drug interactions.

Make sure to read the Drug Facts Label on any over-the-counter product you use, paying close attention to any specific drug interactions that may be listed there.

4. Take any drug interactions involving food and beverages seriously.

Depending on the medications you are taking, your pharmacist or doctor may inquire about specific foods or beverages that you consume. Foods high in vitamin K, for example, are frequently implicated in drug interactions because they can interact with certain blood thinners such as warfarin and make them less effective, perhaps leading to a clot in the blood vessel. Certain citrus juices, such as grapefruit juice, are also well-known for altering the blood levels of certain medications. Calcium can form complexes with some medications, preventing them from being absorbed.

As an example, if you are taking the blood thinner warfarin, raising your vitamin K levels in the body can cause clotting to occur and warfarin to become less effective, perhaps leading to a stroke or heart attack. Beef liver, broccoli, brussel sprouts, cabbage, collard greens, endive, kale, lettuce, mustard greens, parsley, soy beans, spinach, Swiss chard, turnip greens, watercress, and a variety of other vegetables and fruits are high in vitamin K. While it is not necessary to avoid items that contain vitamin K, it is recommended that you consume these products at a constant rate.

Consumption of grapefruit or grapefruit juice may also result in drug interactions, which may increase the level of the medication in your blood, potentially causing drug toxicity, if consumed in excess. Drinking grapefruit juice, for example, might alter the blood levels of some cholesterol-lowering medications known as statins — such as atorvastatin, lovastatin, and simvastatin — and result in severe muscle injury known as rhabdomyolysis, which is a type of kidney failure. Because not all medications in a class of pharmaceuticals, such as statins, may cause an interaction, your doctor will be able to prescribe a different medication to avoid the interaction. In addition to cranberry juice, orange juice, pomegranate juice, and garlic, other foods and beverages might cause medication interactions.

5. Inform your doctor about your caffeine, alcohol, and illegal drug consumption.

Drugs that are commonly used in social situations can have a particularly harsh effect when combined with other drugs. In the case of some asthma medications, such as the beta-2 agonist albuterol (ProAir, Proventil HFA, and Ventolin HFA), this can have a stimulant effect on the body. It is possible that combining albuterol and caffeine will cause sleep disturbances or a high heart rate, which can be problematic in persons who have heart disease. The stimulant impact of caffeine can be additive to the stimulant effect of decongestants such as pseudoephedrine or phenylephrine, as well as vice versa.

The effects of alcohol, particularly when combined with other drugs that cause sedation, can make you more prone to falling or getting into a car accident, putting you at greater risk of injury. Alcohol and opioid pain relievers, as well as anxiety medications such as benzodiazepines, should never be taken together. It is possible to experience life-threatening respiratory depression.

It has been discovered that there is a particularly worrying, though often overlooked, relationship between alcohol and cocaine. In a study published in the journal Addiction, the National Institute on Drug Abuse (NIDA) discovered that the human liver combines cocaine and alcohol to produce a third molecule, cocaethylene, which increases the euphoric effects of cocaine while also increasing the risk of sudden death. According to the National Institute on Drug Abuse, this drug-drug interaction between cocaine and alcohol is a typical two-drug combination that leads to drug-related deaths.

When illicit drugs are coupled with other illicit drugs, the danger is increased significantly. Some injecting drug users use a "speedball," which is a combination of the opioid heroin and cocaine delivered through a single syringe. This combination can be fatal, and it is often used in this manner.

Taking a medication prescribed for someone else is prohibited. Medications are prescribed for a specific individual based on factors such as their age, weight, and specific type of medical condition. As a result of not having a health care practitioner involved while taking pharmaceuticals that have not been prescribed for you, there is no one to check for potential interactions or safety concerns based on your medical circumstances.

A sore throat can be made worse by taking someone else's antibiotic for it. This could not only result in a possible drug interaction, but it could also make your infection worse. It's possible that the antibiotic isn't the best choice for treating the bacterial strain, and that you won't receive the entire course of antibiotics, which can lead to antibiotic resistance and unsuccessful therapy. Furthermore, if your sore throat is caused by a virus rather than a bacterial infection (which is frequently the case), you may not require an antibiotic at all. This is something that your doctor can check for you.

7. Comply with all of the dosing instructions on your prescription bottle.

The directions for taking your medication will be printed on the label of your prescription bottle. For example, you may need to adjust the time intervals between when you take your prescription medications. Some drug interactions are caused by the binding of one medication to another in the stomach. This type of interaction is frequently associated with the use of antacids. Your pharmacist will place a sticker on your bottle to alert you to the possibility of an interaction. In order to avoid the interaction, you may need to space the time of your dosages, taking each medication 2 to 4 hours before or after the other medication.

Antacids can also cause your stomach's pH to rise, which can result in the dissolving of enteric coatings — such as enteric-coated aspirin or ibuprofen — before they should typically dissolve in your intestines. This could result in significant gastrointestinal bleeding or a reduction in the absorption of the medication. Your pharmacist will offer you with precise information on how to proceed.

Do not alter the dosage of your medication unless your doctor has given you permission to do so. If your warning sticker indicates that you should avoid a certain drug or a specific class of drugs altogether, make sure to follow the directions on the label. The use of over-the-counter and prescription medications that may raise the risk of bleeding in patients on blood thinners such as warfarin (ibuprofen, naproxen) or aspirin is recommended for many people taking blood thinners.

8. Inform your health-care provider of any medical conditions you are suffering from.

Oral decongestants available over-the-counter (OTC), such as pseudoephedrine (Sudafed) and phenylephrine (Sudafed PE), can raise your blood pressure. Even if you are on blood pressure medication, this can happen. The use of these drugs should be avoided by people who have uncontrolled or severe high blood pressure (hypertension). You should discuss this interaction with your doctor if you are using blood pressure medications.

Patients suffering from acute angle-closure (narrow-angle) glaucoma, for example, are frequently prescribed the antihistamine diphenhydramine (Benadryl), which has been shown to cause a disease-drug interaction. People who have narrow angles may find that diphenhydramine has anticholinergic effects, which might cause their pupils to dilate and their angle to close. In persons who have angle-closure glaucoma, antihistamines should be avoided, or they should only be administered under the guidance of a physician.

9. Do not purchase medications from untrustworthy online pharmacies.

If you're looking to save money on medications, it's tempting to buy them from untrustworthy websites on the Internet or from countries that may not fully regulate prescription drugs. However, doing so could put your health at risk, whether it's a prescription or over-the-counter medication. According to the United States Food and Drug Administration, "the FDA has not evaluated the safety and effectiveness of imported pharmaceuticals, and the FDA cannot guarantee the identification or potency of these medications."

It is possible that you will receive the incorrect medication, the incorrect strength, or even obsolete or expired prescriptions. If you are unsure of what is in your prescription, you will be unable to do a reliable drug interaction check to rule out any potentially dangerous interactions.

CONCLUSION

Xanax, also known by several generic names, is a benzodiazepine-class psychotropic medication that acts as a short-acting anxiolytic. Xanax, like other benzodiazepines, binds to specific GABAAreceptor sites.

Xanax is a medication that is extensively used and FDA authorized for the medical treatment of panic disorder and anxiety disorders such as generalized anxiety disorder and social anxiety disorder.

Xanax is available in crushed tablet and extended-release capsule formulations for oral use. Anxiolytic, sedative, hypnotic, skeletal muscle relaxant, anticonvulsant, and amnestic characteristics are all found in Xanax.

www.ingramcontent.com/pod-product-compliance
Lightning Source LLC
Chambersburg PA
CBHW050709250726
48662CB00002B/920